‖‖‖ THE STORY OF ‖‖‖
LIN-MANUEL MIRANDA

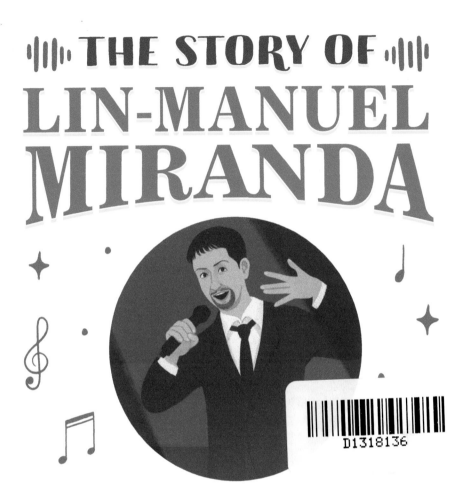

A Biography Book for New Readers

— Written by —
Frank Berrios

— Illustrated by —
Marta Dorado

ROCKRIDGE
PRESS

As a proud Afro-Latino, this book is dedicated to my amazing Puerto Rican family—and all the beautiful Boricuas across the globe. ¡Que viva Puerto Rico!

For general information on our other products and services or to obtain technical support, please contact our Customer Care Department within the United States at (866) 744-2665, or outside the United States at (510) 253-0500.

Rockridge Press publishes its books in a variety of electronic and print formats. Some content that appears in print may not be available in electronic books, and vice versa.

TRADEMARKS: Rockridge Press and the Rockridge Press logo are trademarks or registered trademarks of Callisto Media Inc. and/or its affiliates, in the United States and other countries, and may not be used without written permission. All other trademarks are the property of their respective owners. Rockridge Press is not associated with any product or vendor mentioned in this book.

Series Designer: Angela Navarra

Interior and Cover Designer: Angela Navarra

Art Producer: Hannah Dickerson

Editor: Laura Apperson

Production Editor: Holland Baker

Production Manager: Holly Haydash

Illustrations © 2021 Marta Dorado.

Photography © Joan Marcus/TCD/Prod.DB/Alamy Stock Photo, p. 50; WENN Rights Ltd./ Alamy Stock Photo, p. 52; Joshua Lott/REUTERS/Alamy Stock Photo, p. 53. All maps used under license from Creative Market.

All maps used under license from Creative Market.

Author photo courtesy of Mike Meskin.

Paperback ISBN: 978-1-63807-498-4 | eBook ISBN: 978-1-63878-015-1

R0

CONTENTS

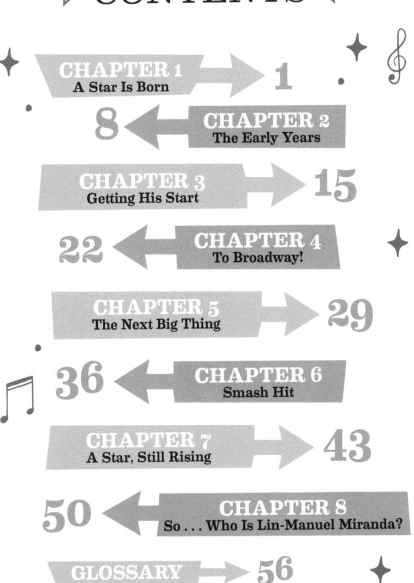

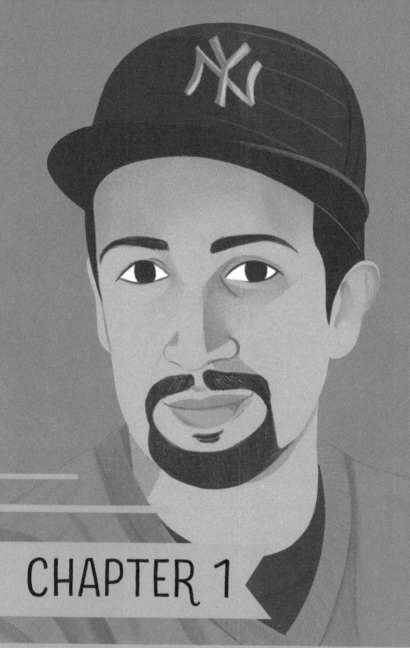

CHAPTER 1

A STAR IS BORN

ᚎ Meet Lin-Manuel Miranda ᚎ

Lin-Manuel Miranda is an award-winning American **composer**, **actor**, **playwright**, **lyricist**, **humanitarian**, **activist**, and proud Puerto Rican. His love of music and movies took him from growing up in the streets of uptown Manhattan to making musicals on Broadway and appearing in Hollywood films! He is the **creator** and original star of the award-winning Broadway musicals *In the Heights* and *Hamilton*. He won a **Pulitzer Prize** for his writing and music in *Hamilton,* and his books have sold over a million copies. He is a cofounder and member of the hip-hop **improv** group Freestyle Love Supreme. He has appeared on television shows including *The Electric Company,* and he's written songs for Disney films like *Moana* and *Encanto*. He was a voice actor on Disney's *DuckTales* and tried to help Big Bird find a new home as a real estate agent on *Sesame*

Street. Lin-Manuel was raised in Inwood, just north of Washington Heights in New York City. As a child, he enjoyed listening to all sorts of music and loved to watch Disney musicals. One of his favorite Disney films was *The Little Mermaid*. In the fourth grade, he memorized and sang a popular song from the film to his entire class. Lin-Manuel was an intelligent and artistic child. Although he seemed to be a born performer, he still had to work hard to achieve his dreams. So, take a seat and get ready to learn more about who Lin-Manuel is, why he was inspired to be an artist, and how he is changing the world!

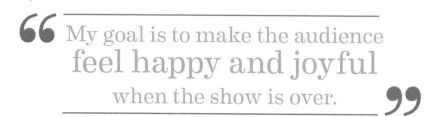

66 My goal is to make the audience feel happy and joyful when the show is over. 99

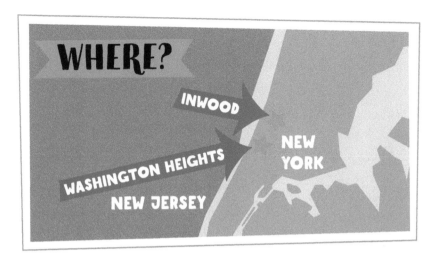

⦀ Lin-Manuel's America ⦀

Lin-Manuel was born in New York City on January 16, 1980. In the 1980s, things like laptops and the internet hadn't yet been invented. Cell phones did exist, but they were as big as bricks and extremely expensive to own. At that time, New York was still recovering from a financial crisis that left many people without jobs. As a result, crime was on the rise across the city. The subway system was in desperate need of upgrades and repairs. Many families struggled to find places to live that weren't too expensive.

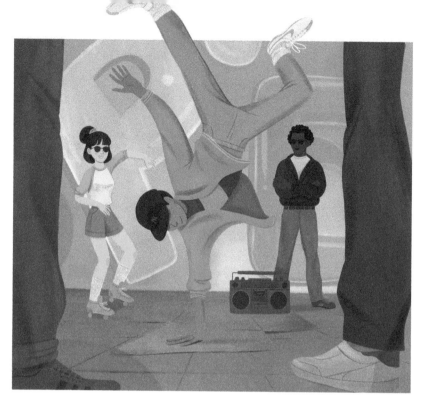

Things were tough, but they weren't all bad. In the 1970s, a new music style called hip-hop had spread through the boroughs of New York. Created by young African American, Caribbean, and Latino, or Latinx, Americans, this music spoke about the triumphs and troubles that many people of color faced every day. Around the same time, the sounds of salsa music by Latin artists like Rubén Blades, Celia Cruz, and Héctor Lavoe could be heard all over the city.

Lin-Manuel's parents, Luz Towns-Miranda and Luis A. Miranda Jr., were both **Boricuas** (boh-REE-kwahs), an affectionate term for Puerto Ricans which pays tribute to the island's original people, the Taíno. Puerto Ricans proudly embrace the Taíno, African, and Spanish influences in their culture. Puerto Rico is an island in the Caribbean that is a commonwealth

JUMP –IN THE– THINK TANK

Lin-Manuel is proud of his Puerto Rican **heritage**. Do you know your family history? Ask a family member to share some stories so you can write them down!

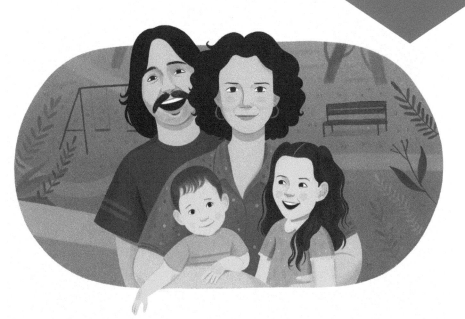

of the United States. That means Puerto Ricans are citizens of the United States. Unfortunately, Puerto Ricans who live on the island don't have the same rights as other Americans. They can join the military, but they are not allowed to vote. They also don't have a representative in Congress. Many Puerto Ricans decided to leave the island to come to the mainland United States in search of more opportunities, like better-paying jobs and bigger schools.

WHEN?

A new style of Latin music called salsa is created.

Hip-hop emerges in New York City.

Lin-Manuel is born in New York City on January 16.

1960s — **1970s** — **1980**

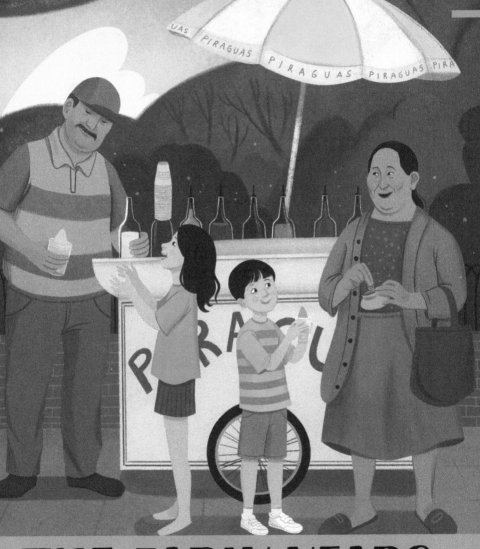

CHAPTER 2

THE EARLY YEARS

⫻ **Growing Up in New York City** ⫻

Lin-Manuel's father, Luis A. Miranda Jr., was born in Vega Alta, Puerto Rico. At eighteen, he came to New York for graduate school, even though he spoke little English. He soon met another Puerto Rican student named Luz Towns. Luz had a daughter, also named Luz. The two students fell in love and married in 1978. Luis adopted little Luz, and in 1980, Lin-Manuel was born. Lin-Manuel and his sister had a **nanny** named Edmunda Claudio. Lin-Manuel affectionately called her *Abuela* (ah-BWEH-lah), which means "grandmother" in Spanish, even though she wasn't his actual grandmother.

Growing up, Lin-Manuel seemed to live in two worlds. In his mostly Latino neighborhood, almost everyone spoke Spanish. Owners of the little **bodegas**, or corner stores, knew exactly how customers liked their coffee. Lin-Manuel and Luz would enjoy colorful ***piraguas*** (pee-RAH-gwahs), treats made of shaved ice and flavored syrup. But when he went to school, Lin-Manuel rode a yellow bus to Hunter College Elementary School in the wealthy Upper East Side neighborhood. It was a good school, but only a few students were Latino like Lin-Manuel. He often felt like an outsider.

Thankfully, Lin-Manuel spent summers with family in Puerto Rico. It was a wonderful way for him to reconnect with his culture. His family introduced Lin-Manuel and Luz to many

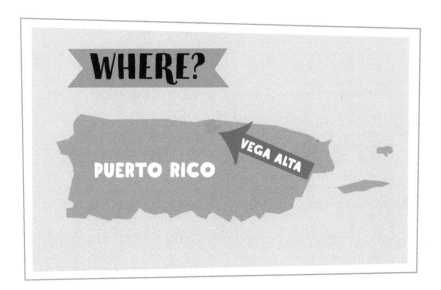

WHERE?

PUERTO RICO

VEGA ALTA

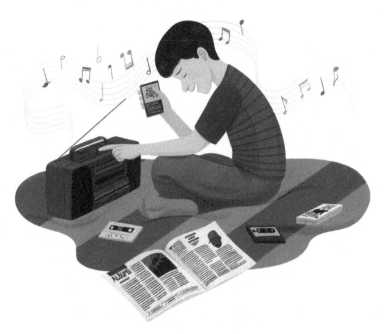

styles of music, including salsa, because they loved to dance! They also enjoyed listening to **cast albums** of musicals. Luz took Lin-Manuel to see early hip-hop films like *Beat Street,* and he would often steal her cassette tapes so he could learn the lyrics to his favorite rap songs!

A Natural Performer

New York City is famous for its many theaters where people can see plays and musicals. Most of these theaters are in the Theater District in

Midtown Manhattan, commonly referred to as Broadway, which was only a short subway ride away from Inwood. In 1987, when Lin-Manuel was just seven years old, his parents took him to see a musical called *Les Misérables*. He spotted a child in the cast and was jealous! He wondered how a kid his age was able to find a job onstage.

The Miranda Family

LUIS A. MIRANDA JR.
1954–PRESENT

LUZ TOWNS-MIRANDA
1951–PRESENT

VANESSA NADAL
1982–PRESENT

LIN-MANUEL MIRANDA
1980–PRESENT

LUZ MIRANDA-CRESPO
C. 1974–PRESENT

SEBASTIAN MIRANDA
2014–PRESENT

FRANCISCO MIRANDA
2018–PRESENT

JUMP
—IN THE—
THINK TANK

Lin-Manuel enjoys being onstage and making people laugh. Do you like to perform? If so, share your talents with other people!

Lin-Manuel took piano lessons and started composing his own music and filming movies for school projects. But his life changed when he saw the film *The Little Mermaid* in 1989. He dragged his family back to see it again and again. His favorite character was Sebastian the crab.

Lin-Manuel was a quick thinker who was known around school for making people laugh. In the sixth grade, he landed the role of rock star Conrad Birdie in a school production of *Bye Bye Birdie*. Not long after, he decided that he would be an actor.

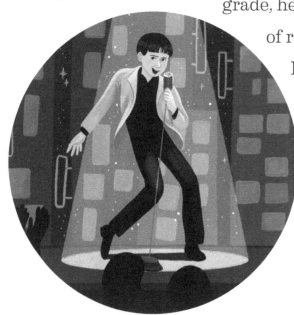

During his senior year at Hunter College High School, Lin-Manuel met Stephen Sondheim. Stephen Sondheim was an award-winning composer who wrote the lyrics for *West Side Story,* one of Lin-Manuel's favorite musicals. Sondheim shared stories that continue to influence and inspire Lin-Manuel to this day. Later in his senior year at Hunter, Lin-Manuel went on to direct a production of *West Side Story*. Hip-hop also continued to loom large in Lin-Manuel's life. He began to follow and study a wide variety of artists like Queen Latifah and Big Pun.

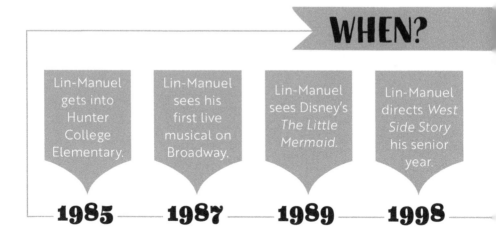

WHEN?

Lin-Manuel gets into Hunter College Elementary.

Lin-Manuel sees his first live musical on Broadway.

Lin-Manuel sees Disney's *The Little Mermaid.*

Lin-Manuel directs *West Side Story* his senior year.

1985 — **1987** — **1989** — **1998**

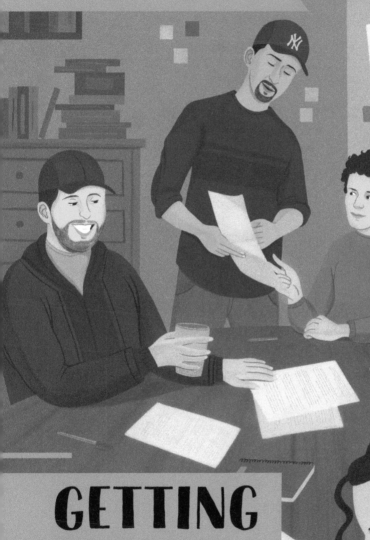
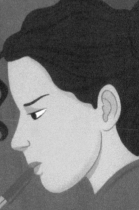
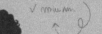
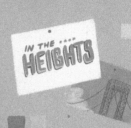

CHAPTER 3

GETTING HIS START

ᐧ|ᐧ Talent and Smarts ᐧ|ᐧ

After high school in 1998, Lin-Manuel studied theater and film at Wesleyan University in Connecticut. Growing up, Lin-Manuel was often the only Puerto Rican in his class, and most of his school friends were white. The same was true when he arrived at Wesleyan, but while there Lin-Manuel lived in a Latino program house where he became friends with other Latino students. Like him, they grew up speaking Spanish at home and English in school. For the first time, Lin-Manuel had friends who shared his life experience. They understood how it felt to straddle two worlds.

> **"** I grew up and live in one of the most musical neighborhoods in New York. This is a world where bodies in the street sing, sweat, and dance. **"**

During his second year at Wesleyan, Lin-Manuel began writing and composing a musical called *In the Heights*. He drew inspiration from the people and places he knew from his childhood and from the experiences of his new college friends. For the first time, Lin-Manuel was telling stories that were close to his heart. His one-act version of *In the Heights* was an instant hit with his classmates. He wondered if it could someday be a Broadway play.

Around the same time, Lin-Manuel's father cocreated a **bilingual** newspaper called *Manhattan Times*, reporting on issues facing the Latino community in upper Manhattan. During the summer, Lin-Manuel researched and wrote columns for the newspaper. His work there opened his eyes to the wonderful diversity of his community and many of the common issues they faced. In 2002, Lin-Manuel graduated from Wesleyan and decided to return home to Inwood.

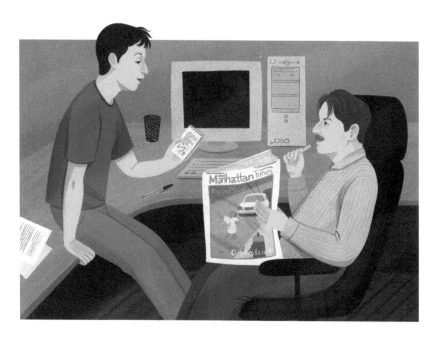

He wasn't exactly sure what his future would hold, but he was eager to find out.

⫾⫾⫾ Back in the Big Apple ⫾⫾⫾

Lin-Manuel was happy to be back in his old neighborhood, but he struggled to figure out his next move. At first he taught seventh-grade English as a substitute teacher at Hunter Elementary, where he'd gone to school as a child.

JUMP -IN THE- THINK TANK

Lin-Manuel always loved his neighborhood. What do you like about the neighborhood you live in? Is there anything you dislike, or want to change?

He loved the job, but he missed the excitement of writing songs and performing on stage. Eventually, Lin-Manuel was offered a full-time job at Hunter Elementary as a teacher. After asking his father for advice, Lin-Manuel decided to turn down the job to pursue his dream of writing musicals. Around this time, he also reconnected with a friend he knew from high school named Vanessa. They dated and fell in love!

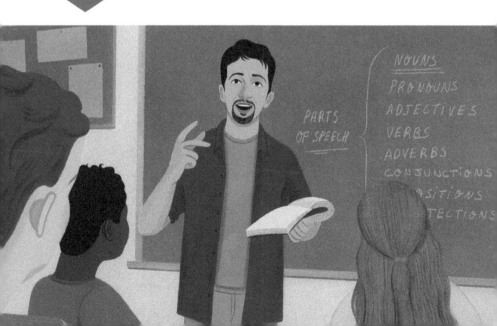

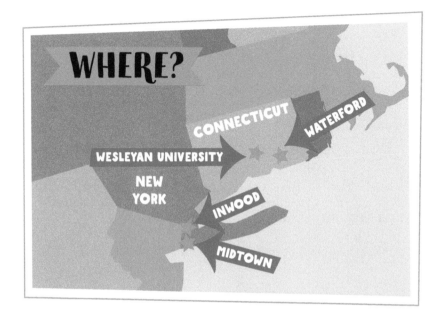

Lin-Manuel kept working on *In the Heights,* with many **collaborators**. Tommy Kail had been producing plays in the basement of a small bookstore with several other former Wesleyan students. Lin-Manuel would pop into the bookstore to share new scenes, characters, and ideas for *In the Heights* with Tommy. Lin introduced Tommy to Bill Sherman, another graduate of Wesleyan. Bill had a degree in music and was a huge fan of hip-hop. When Lin and Bill needed someone to arrange songs, they turned to composer Alex Lacamoire. Meanwhile, Lin continued to do more research, revise storylines, and add new songs to the play. After finding **producers**, Lin-Manuel worked with a playwright named Quiara Alegría Hudes, who wrote the nonmusical parts of the play, also known as the "book."

After a quick run at the Eugene O'Neill Theater Center in Waterford, Connecticut, *In the Heights* made its **off-Broadway** debut in 2007 at the 37 Arts Theatre in New York City. Little did Lin-Manuel know it would forever change his life!

WHEN?

2000	2002	2005	2007
Lin-Manuel performs *In the Heights* at Wesleyan University.	Lin-Manuel graduates from Wesleyan University.	Lin-Manuel reconnects with future wife Vanessa Nadal.	*In the Heights* debuts off-Broadway.

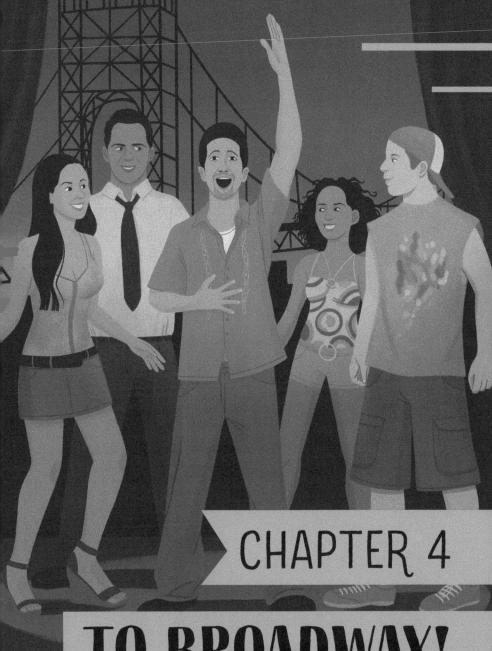

CHAPTER 4

TO BROADWAY!

⫙⫙ Sweet Success ⫙⫙

Audiences were impressed by what they saw and heard at performances of *In the Heights*. Lin-Manuel included hip-hop, a heavy dose of salsa, and a few traditional Broadway ballads in the music. The combination was a hit with audience members both young and old! They were especially taken with Lin-Manuel's performance as the main character, a friendly bodega owner named Usnavi who learns he has sold a winning lottery ticket to someone in the neighborhood.

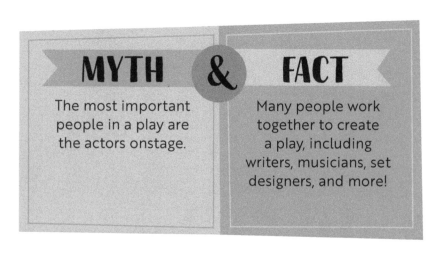

MYTH & FACT

The most important people in a play are the actors onstage.

Many people work together to create a play, including writers, musicians, set designers, and more!

With its hopeful messages of family, love, community, and home, positive reviews quickly followed the first few performances.

JUMP
–IN THE–
THINK
TANK

Do you like to act, dance, and sing? If so, put on a play! Work with your friends to write a story and have fun!

It takes a lot of people to produce and stage even the smallest play. It also takes time and, sometimes, a lot of money. Lin-Manuel was lucky to find good people to work with, like Tommy, Bill, Quiara, and Alex. They also found producers who trusted and believed in their talent and vision. Lin-Manuel, Tommy, and Quiara used the off-Broadway run to figure out what needed to be fixed in the show. They met and exchanged ideas for hours after each performance. They tweaked dialogue every day, revised and rewrote songs, and even cut characters when necessary. The goal was to make the play the very best it could be, and that meant long nights at the theater. With six shows a week, Lin-Manuel was constantly working. He often slept on a couch at the rehearsal space instead of going home to get rest in his own bed.

ᛁᛁᛁ A Star Rising ᛁᛁᛁ

Eventually, word of the new, exciting off-Broadway play *In the Heights* spread through both the arts and Latino communities.

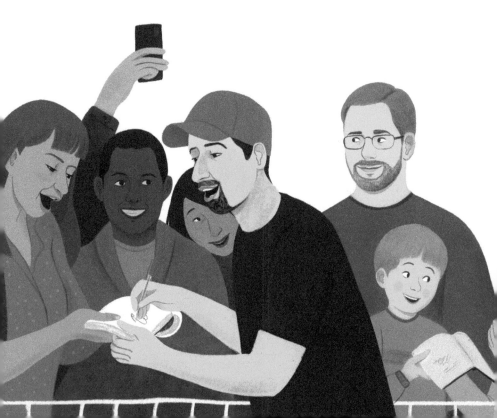

In the Heights was a hit! Lin-Manuel and the rest of the team prepared to move to a bigger theater. A Broadway theater, which has 500 or more seats, is much harder to fill than an off-Broadway theater, which can have as few as 100 seats. The producers decided to advertise the new Broadway show by shooting a commercial where the show was set—in Washington Heights! The cast enjoyed performing on the actual city streets in front of the people who had inspired Lin-Manuel to write the show.

The success of *In the Heights* changed Lin-Manuel's life. Suddenly, people recognized him wherever he went. He gave autographs to fans after performances. *In the Heights* wasn't only a hit with fans—critics loved it, too! The play won a Tony Award, which is the highest award a live show on Broadway can achieve. The cast album for the musical won a Grammy Award, an award that recognizes achievements in music.

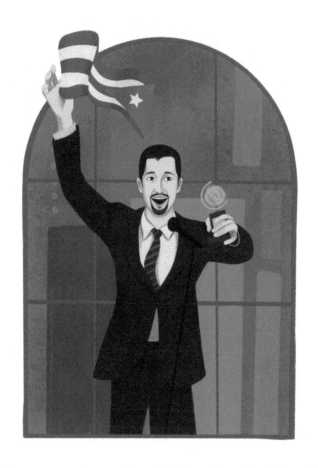

The play was also a finalist for the Pulitzer Prize for Drama, a huge honor!

Most Broadway shows swap out actors after about a year to give them a rest, and also to allow new talent to flourish and grow. After a year as the character Usnavi, Lin-Manuel decided to take a break to pursue other opportunities. Thankfully,

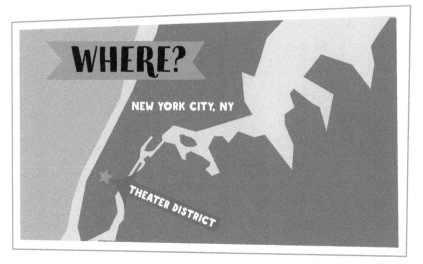

the show continued to be extremely successful without him. More importantly, Lin-Manuel was about to work on something new—something that would be much, much bigger than anything he could have ever imagined!

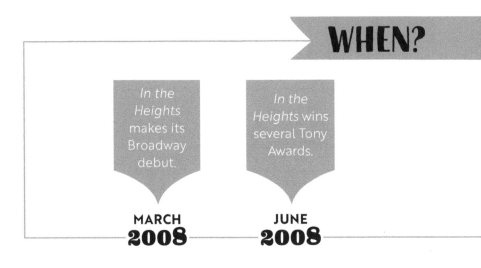

WHEN?

In the Heights makes its Broadway debut.

In the Heights wins several Tony Awards.

MARCH
2008

JUNE
2008

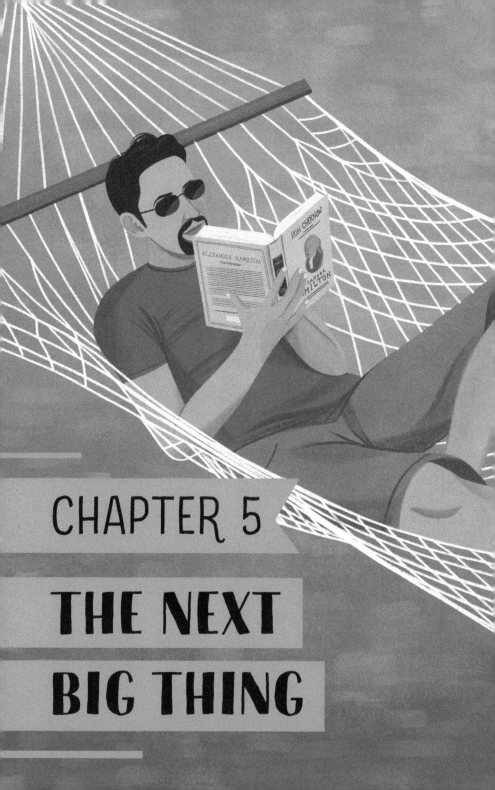

CHAPTER 5

THE NEXT BIG THING

The Book that Changed ᛁᛁᛁ Everything ᛁᛁᛁ

In 2008, Lin-Manuel went to Mexico on vacation. He brought along a **biography** of Alexander Hamilton written by Ron Chernow. Hamilton was one of the lesser-known **Founding Fathers** of the United States. His journey, from poor **immigrant** to one of the builders of our nation, felt both unique and familiar to Lin-Manuel. Like Alexander Hamilton, Lin-Manuel's father, Luis, had come to New York alone as a young student. The two men were both interested and involved in the politics of their day. Hamilton's rags-to-riches story also mirrored the lives of some of Lin-Manuel's favorite rappers, like Run-DMC and The Notorious B.I.G. Lin-Manuel came up with an idea for a hip-hop project based on the book. It would be called *The Hamilton Mixtape*.

When he came home from vacation, Lin-Manuel invited Ron Chernow, the author of *Alexander Hamilton*, to see *In the Heights*. After the show, Lin-Manuel told Ron about *The Hamilton Mixtape*. Ron agreed to work with him as a **consultant** on the new project. Lin-Manuel worked on the Hamilton project while taking on other projects as well, including working with Stephen Sondheim to write Spanish-language dialogue for the Broadway revival of West Side Story.

In 2009, Lin-Manuel was invited to perform a song from *In the Heights* at the White House. Instead, he performed a rap about Alexander Hamilton. As the audience—which included President Barack Obama, First Lady Michelle Obama, and their daughters—looked on,

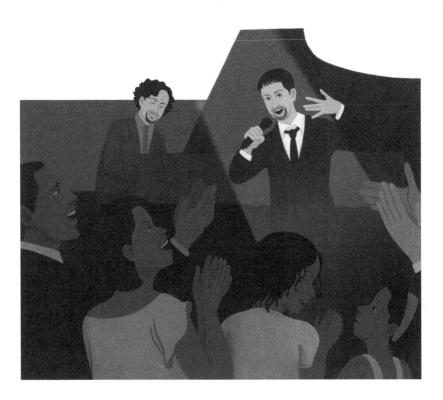

Lin-Manuel laid down a few rhymes that would one day become part of the groundbreaking musical *Hamilton*.

ᴵᴵᴵ *The Hamilton Mixtape* ᴵᴵᴵ

Lin-Manuel was encouraged by the positive response at the White House. But two years passed before he was confident enough to share the next song. One very exciting life event happened while he was writing, though. In 2010, Lin-Manuel married Vanessa, the love of his life!

In 2011, during a benefit show for a Manhattan theater, Lin-Manuel was finally ready to share a second song from *The Hamilton Mixtape*, "My Shot." Once again, the crowd went wild! Tommy Kail also thought it was great. But two songs in two years was very slow. He asked Lin-Manuel to write faster.

A few days later, Lincoln Center invited Lin-Manuel to perform in the American Songbook concert series. The event would be on January 11, 2012, Alexander Hamilton's 255th birthday. Lin-Manuel prepared twelve songs from *The Hamilton Mixtape*. Even though the Founding Fathers were all white men, the songs Lin-Manuel wrote would need to be performed

 The hardest part of working is finding collaborators you can trust.

by skillful rappers. Most of the actors he chose were people of color. That night, fans and critics alike—including some of the biggest names in theater—were blown away by his work! The incredible reaction from the audience helped Lin-Manuel secure a producer for *The Hamilton Mixtape*. In 2013, an electrifying performance at Vassar College set the stage for an off-Broadway premiere of the musical.

As the writer and main character of the show, Lin-Manuel was prepared for long rehearsal days.

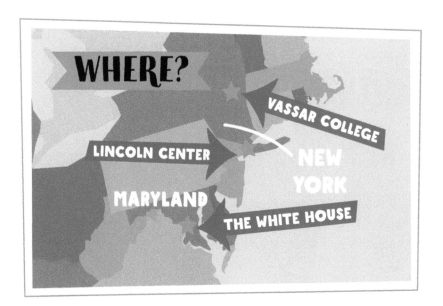

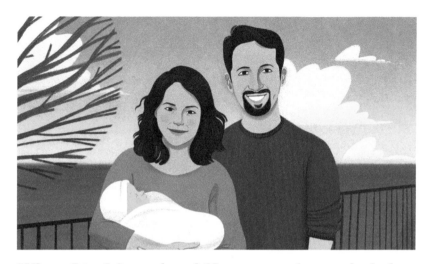

When Lin-Manuel and Vanessa welcomed a baby boy to the family in November 2014, it gave him the extra boost of energy needed to prepare for the off-Broadway debut of *Hamilton: An American Musical* on January 20, 2015, at the Public Theater.

WHEN?

Lin-Manuel marries Vanessa.	Lin-Manuel performs parts of *The Hamilton Mixtape.*	Sebastian, Lin-Manuel's first son, is born.	*Hamilton* makes its off-Broadway debut
2010	**2012**	**2014**	**2015**

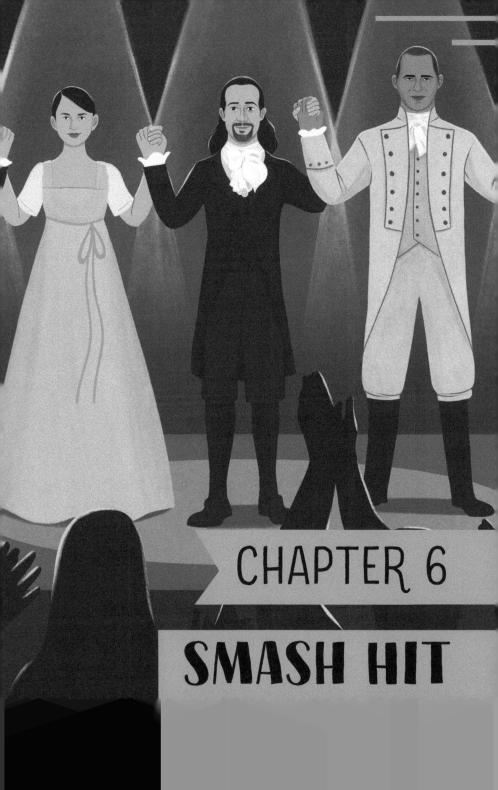

CHAPTER 6

SMASH HIT

⑪ Back to Broadway ⑪

Hamilton's off-Broadway debut was a runaway
smash! After just three months, it was decided
that the musical would move to Broadway. As
word of mouth spread, tickets became harder
and harder to buy. Because Broadway tickets
are often very expensive, Lin-Manuel created
Ham4Ham, a lottery that allowed people to see
the show for ten dollars—the bill that bears
Alexander Hamilton's face.

Lin-Manuel wanted to throw open the doors to
musical theater and create new roles for people
who looked, talked, and walked like him. Instead
of casting only white characters, Lin-Manuel
found new talent in people of color. The casting
had a huge impact on the success of the show.
Lin-Manuel placed a diverse cast on the stage,
and performers of color rejoiced at the chance
to play roles they otherwise would have never
been offered.

MYTH	&	FACT
Lin-Manuel became a star overnight.		Lin-Manuel worked hard for many years as both a writer and an actor before he became a big star.

The show was an instant success and helped spark conversations about the positive role of immigrants in America. Ron Chernow's biography of Alexander Hamilton once again became popular as people wanted to learn more about the Founding Father's life. Lin-Manuel also cowrote a book which included lyrics from the show alongside details about his creative process. The book became an instant bestseller! In addition to rave reviews, *Hamilton* won the Pulitzer Prize for Drama and earned a record-breaking sixteen Tony nominations! The show went on to win eleven Tony Awards,

Lin-Manuel loved to sing and act as a child. Now that's his full-time job. Find something you like to do, then figure out how to make it a career!

including two for Lin-Manuel himself. The cast album also won a Grammy award.

From Stage ·|||· to Camera ·|||·

Performing eight plays a week can be tough, so less than a year after the Broadway debut of *Hamilton,* Lin-Manuel decided to stop acting in the show. Because everyone knew who he was, it wasn't long before movie producers and directors wanted to work with him. Lin-Manuel was never shy about sharing his love of Disney films as a child. So when Disney approached him about a new movie called *Moana,* he leapt at the chance to work with them. Lin-Manuel wrote songs and composed lyrics for the film, including "You're

Welcome," sung by Dwayne "The Rock" Johnson. The animated film was an instant hit with moviegoers of all ages! The next year, one of the songs he had written for the film was nominated for an Oscar. Although he didn't win the award, Lin-Manuel was proud to have been nominated. Plus, he got to take his mother to the awards ceremony! It was a night they would never forget.

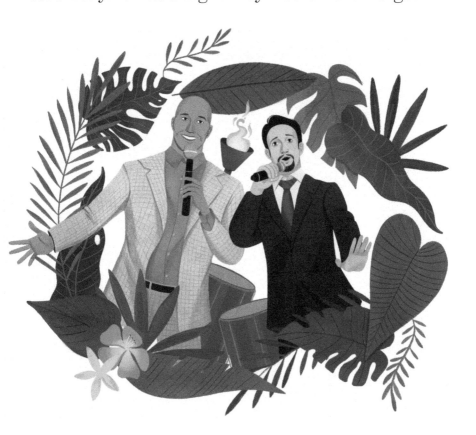

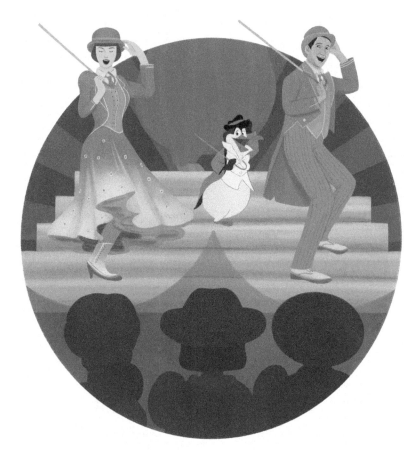

Lin-Manuel was also excited to take on
the role of Jack the Lamplighter in the *Mary
Poppins Returns* feature film. On the film set of
Mary Poppins Returns, Lin-Manuel didn't have
to worry about every detail of the project. He
simply had to focus on singing, dancing, and

acting, which he did very well. He earned a Golden Globe nomination for his performance in the film!

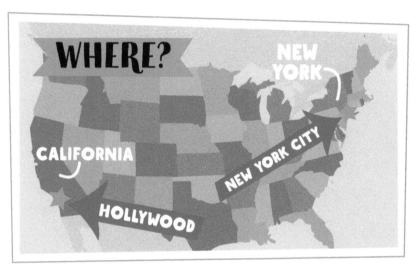

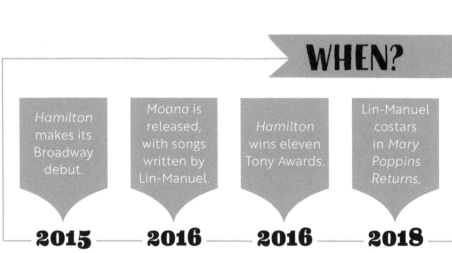

WHEN?

Hamilton makes its Broadway debut.	*Moana* is released, with songs written by Lin-Manuel.	*Hamilton* wins eleven Tony Awards.	Lin-Manuel costars in *Mary Poppins Returns*.
2015	**2016**	**2016**	**2018**

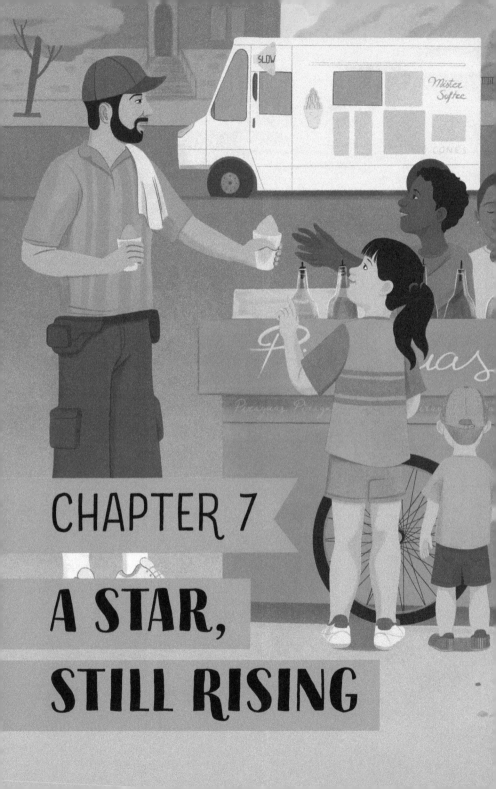

CHAPTER 7

A STAR, STILL RISING

‖‖ Looking toward the Future ‖‖

Lin-Manuel released daily greetings via Twitter to keep in touch with fans in 2018 after he and Vanessa welcomed Francisco, their second child, to the family. Later that year, his tweets were collected, illustrated, and published as *Gmorning, Gnight!: Little Pep Talks for Me & You,* which became a bestseller! That same year, Lin-Manuel, Thomas Kail, Andy Blankenbuehler, and Alex Lacamoire received a Kennedy Center Honors award for their work on *Hamilton.*

Lin-Manuel's ties to Puerto Rico are strong. After Hurricane Maria damaged homes and destroyed roads on the island in 2017, Lin-Manuel wanted

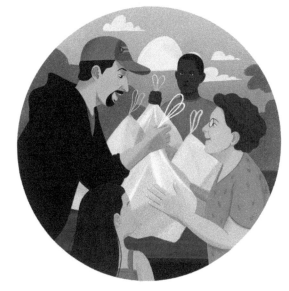

Lin-Manuel inspires people with his work and kind words. Is there something you can do or say to make someone's day a little brighter?

to help his fellow Boricuas rebuild. He donated money to charities and traveled to the island to pass out food and water. He also donated money to the University of Puerto Rico to renovate their damaged theater. To raise even more money and awareness, he brought *Hamilton* to Puerto Rico in 2019. He even resumed the lead role! In just three weeks, he raised nearly $15 million for arts organizations across the island.

Also in 2019, the film version of *In the Heights* began shooting **on location** in Washington Heights. Lin-Manuel felt he was too old to play the role of Usnavi, so he decided to play the Piragua Guy, a slightly older character with a smaller role. The film was released in 2021 and it was a huge success! While the film cast many Latino actors, it also received criticism for not featuring enough **Afro-Latinos** in lead roles, despite Washington Heights being home to many Afro-Latino people. Lin-Manuel acknowledged the misstep and vowed to do better in the future. The year before, in 2020, the *Hamilton* film, which featured the original cast, aired on Disney+. In 2021, Lin-Manuel provided the voice of the lead character in *Vivo*, an animated film about a musical monkey, and he worked on the live action version of *The Little Mermaid*. It was a dream come true to work on a remake of his favorite film.

An American Legacy

Lin-Manuel felt lucky to have been born in New York City in the 1980s. His Puerto Rican parents exposed him to the New York art scene at an early age. It allowed him to imagine himself in those worlds—in the movies, on the

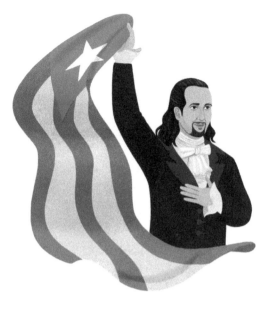

stage—dancing, singing, and acting! His sister introduced him to hip-hop, which would go on to influence how he talked, thought, and dressed. His love of both Latino and New York culture, as well as American history, led him to write plays which will have a lasting impact in theater and beyond. *Hamilton* continues to be one of the most popular Broadway shows of all time. It has introduced the world to a talented group of new stars who have gone on to thrive beyond the stage. *Hamilton* has also had an impact in the classroom. The Hamilton Education Program aims to improve how children learn about American history.

> **"** I come from a family of really **hard workers. My parents** worked the entire time we were growing up. I think my parents inspired that in us ... even when we're having fun we have to feel productive. **"**

When he first came up with the idea for *Hamilton,* Lin-Manuel wasn't sure if people would pay to watch a Broadway musical about Alexander Hamilton. He didn't know if using hip-hop to tell that story would be well received. Thankfully, his family and friends encouraged him to follow his dreams and work hard. Along the way, he made many sacrifices and difficult decisions about how to express himself as an artist. In the end, the long hours paid off. Lin-Manuel is doing what he loves to do— entertaining people all over the world!

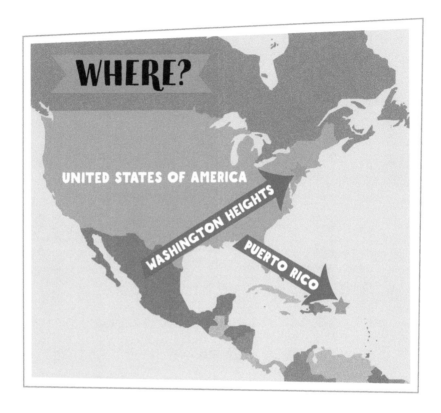

WHERE?

UNITED STATES OF AMERICA

WASHINGTON HEIGHTS

PUERTO RICO

WHEN?

2018	2019	2020	2021
Lin-Manuel's second son, Francisco, is born.	Lin-Manuel performs *Hamilton* for charity in Puerto Rico.	*Hamilton* film is released.	*In the Heights* and *Vivo* films are released.

CHAPTER 8

SO . . . WHO IS LIN-MANUEL MIRANDA?

?

||| Challenge Accepted! |||

Now that you know so much about Lin-Manuel Miranda's amazing accomplishments, let's test your knowledge with a little who, what, when, where, why, and how quiz. Feel free to look back in the text to find the answers if you need to, but try to remember first.

1 Who is Lin-Manuel Miranda?

→ A A writer
→ B An actor
→ C A composer and lyricist
→ D All of the above

2 What year was Lin-Manuel born?

→ A 1980
→ B 1982
→ C 1985
→ D 1988

3 **Where was Lin-Manuel born?**

→ A Middletown, Connecticut

→ B New York, New York

→ C Vega Alta, Puerto Rico

→ D Los Angeles, California

4 **Lin-Manuel's parents came from which island nation in the Caribbean?**

→ A The Dominican Republic

→ B Cuba

→ C Jamaica

→ D Puerto Rico

5 **What is the name of Lin-Manuel's favorite character from *The Little Mermaid*?**

→ A Ariel

→ B Flounder

→ C Sebastian

→ D Scuttle

6 **Lin-Manuel wrote a play about which Founding Father?**

A Alexander Hamilton

B Benjamin Franklin

C George Washington

D John Jay

7 **From which university did Lin-Manuel graduate?**

A University of Puerto Rico

B New York University

C Wesleyan University

D Hunter College

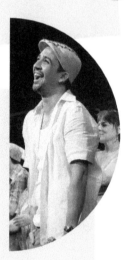

8 **Why did Lin-Manuel write *In the Heights*?**

A He wanted to write a play about the neighborhood he grew up in.

B He wanted to write a play with positive Latino role models.

C He wanted to create more roles for actors of all colors.

D All of the above.

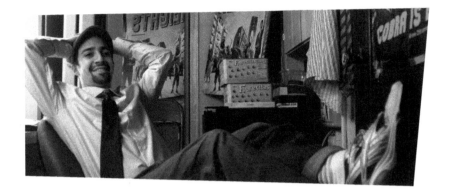

9 **Who wrote the biography which inspired Lin-Manuel to write a play about Alexander Hamilton?**

→ A Barack Obama

→ B Ron Chernow

→ C Stephen Sondheim

→ D Tommy Kail

10 **Lin-Manuel has appeared in which of the following?**

→ A Broadway

→ B Movies

→ C Television shows

→ D All of the above

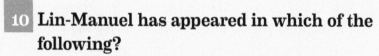

ᵢ||ᵢ **Our World** ᵢ||ᵢ

Lin-Manuel's dedication to telling stories in
his unique way has had a lasting impact on the
world of entertainment. His work on Broadway
laid the groundwork for a successful career, not
just for himself but for many others! He also
proved that musicals could appeal to a wide
range of people.

→ Lin-Manuel made history cool! Writing a play about
one of the Founding Fathers has encouraged students to
understand that learning about history can be fun and
relatable to our current everyday lives.

→ By casting people of color in a wide variety of roles,
Lin-Manuel changed the look of Broadway! Many Latino,
Black, and Asian actors struggled to find roles before
Lin-Manuel arrived on the scene. His decision to cast
nonwhite actors allowed others to "think outside the box"
and consider a wider variety of talent for their shows.

→ Lin-Manuel used hip-hop and salsa to change the
sound of Broadway! By adding new styles of music to
the traditional musical, Lin-Manuel injected energy
and excitement into an industry that some thought was
struggling to survive.

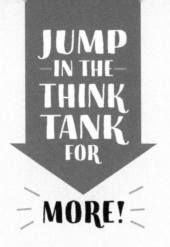

JUMP IN THE THINK TANK FOR

MORE!

Lin-Manuel always liked to entertain people and make them laugh. But he had to work hard to become a star! He wasn't always sure his dreams would come true, but thankfully, he never gave up!

→ Lin-Manuel's love of music, history, and culture led him to the Broadway stage. What kind of music do you enjoy? Can you play an instrument or sing? If so, start a band with some friends!

→ Family and friends have always been important to Lin-Manuel. Do you like to play games or watch movies with your family or friends? What else do you enjoy doing together?

→ To raise money after Hurricane Maria, Lin-Manuel brought his *Hamilton* play to Puerto Rico. He wanted to help Puerto Rico financially by bringing tourists back to the island. What can you do to help someone or make something better in your home, school, or community?

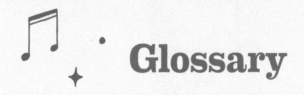

Glossary

activist: A person who works to bring about change for something they care very much about

actor: A person who performs as a character onstage or on the screen

Afro-Latino: A Latino person who recognizes and identifies with their African ancestors

bilingual: To write or speak in two languages

biography: A person's life story

bodega: A small grocery store, usually located on the corner of a city block, found mainly in urban Latino communities

Boricua: An affectionate term for Puerto Ricans which pays tribute to the island's original people, the Taíno

cast album: A recording of the songs from a musical

collaborator: A person who works with others on a project

composer: A person who writes music, especially as their job

consultant: A person who gives advice on a project

creator: The person who comes up with an idea for a story

Founding Fathers: The leaders who united the thirteen colonies, led them in their fight for independence from England, and established a government for the new US.

heritage: The people, traditions, customs, and history of the place of a person's birth and/or their descendants

humanitarian: A person who works to help everyone have better lives

immigrant: A person born in one country who moves to another country and settles there

improv: An exercise where artists, like actors or dancers, create a performance on the spot without rehearsals

lyricist: A person who writes the words to a song

nanny: A person whose job it is to care for children

off-Broadway: A smaller theater located outside of the main Broadway Theater District

on location: Filmed in the area where the story takes place

piragua: A Puerto Rican treat of shaved ice and flavored syrup

playwright: A person who writes a play

producer: The person who raises money and keeps track of spending for a TV show, movie, or play

Pulitzer Prize: An important prize given to American writers

Bibliography

Broadway.com Staff. "Stars on Sondheim: Lin-Manuel Miranda on the Sondheim Email He Framed." Broadway.com. March 22, 2020. Broadway.com/buzz/198860/stars-on-sondheim-lin-manuel-miranda-on-the-sondheim-email-he-framed/

Feinstein, Mara. "Lin-Manuel Miranda Opens Up about Fatherhood, *In the Heights*, and Why He Answers Every Fan Letter." Paper Magazine. June 18, 2021. Parade.com/1221102/maramovies/lin-manuel-miranda-in-the-heights/

Fernández, Alexia; Russian, Ale. "Lin Manuel's Dad Predicted Son's Fame." People Magazine. October 7, 2020. People.com/movies/lin-manuel-mirandas-dad-luis-predicted-his-fame/

Gilder Lehrman Institute of American History. Hamilton Education Program. Hamilton.GilderLehrman.org. 2021. GilderLehrman.org/programs-and-events/hamilton-education-program

Manners, Ivette. "Lin-Manuel Miranda's Family Takes Center Stage." New York Lifestyle Magazine. 2016. NewYorkLifestylesMagazine.com/articles/2016/05/linmanuel.html

Maranzani, Barbara. "How Lin-Manuel Miranda's Childhood Inspired 'In the Heights.'" Biography.com. June 7, 2021. Biography.com/news/lin-manuel-miranda-in-the-heights-inspiration

Miranda, Lin-Manuel. Official Website. LinManuel.com. 2020. LinManuel.com

Miranda, Lin-Manuel; Hudes, Quiara Alegría; McCarter, Jeremy. *In the Heights: Finding Home*. New York. Random House, an imprint and a division of Penguin Random House LLC, 2015.

Miranda, Lin-Manuel; McCarter, Jeremy. *Hamilton: The Revolution*. New York. Grand Central Publishing, a division of Hachette Book Group, Inc., 2016.

Tsioulcas, Anastasia. "Lin-Manuel Miranda Apologizes for lack of Afro-Latinx Actors in 'In the Heights.'" NPR.org. June 15, 2021. NPR.org/2021/06/15/1006606967/lin-manuel-miranda-apologizes-for-lack-of-afro-latinx-actors-in-in-the-heights

WienerElementary.org. Musician of the Week, Lin-Manuel Miranda. 2020. WeinerElementary.org/lin-manuel-miranda.html

Acknowledgments

As Luis A. Miranda, Jr. once said, "Country and family are the most important things in life." With that in mind, I would like to acknowledge Boricuas around the world. Puerto Ricans proudly come in all shapes, sizes, and colors—which is a lesson that should be embraced everywhere. Love is love is love is love! I would also like to acknowledge all of my amazing ancestors—their love, sacrifice, and guidance always gives me the strength to keep moving forward. *¡Siempre pa'lante!*

About the Author

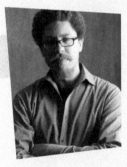

Frank Berrios is a Puerto Rican writer born in Spanish Harlem, New York City. He is the author of *The Story of Joe Biden*, *The Story of Stan Lee*, and *The Story of Misty Copeland*, as well as *Jackie Robinson*, *Miles Morales: Spider-Man*, *Football with Dad*, and *Soccer with Mom* in the *Little Golden Book* series. Learn more about his work at FrankBerriosBooks.com.

About the Illustrator

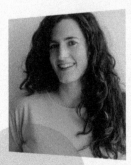

Marta Dorado is a full-time freelance illustrator born in Gijón (Asturias, Spain) in 1989 and raised in a nearby village. She attended university in Pamplona, where she still lives, and started a career as a graphic designer in the advertising industry. Marta's childhood, surrounded by nature and close to the sea, strongly influences her work.

WHO WILL INSPIRE YOU NEXT?

EXPLORE A WORLD OF HEROES AND ROLE MODELS IN ***THE STORY OF...*** BIOGRAPHY SERIES FOR NEW READERS.

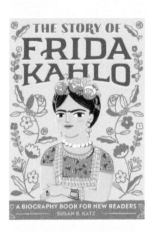

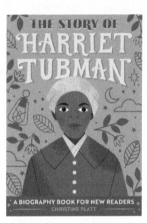

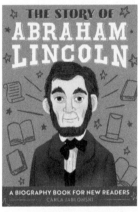

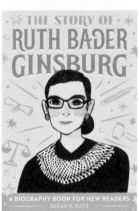

LOOK FOR THIS SERIES
WHEREVER BOOKS AND EBOOKS ARE SOLD

Alexander Hamilton	Jane Goodall
Albert Einstein	Barack Obama
Martin Luther King Jr.	Helen Keller
George Washington	Marie Curie

CPSIA information can be obtained
at www.ICGtesting.com
Printed in the USA
JSHW030516150322
23789JS00004B/6